Congratulations on choosing this Semi-Permanent Brow Training Programme—an immersive journey into the artistry and precision of enhancing natural beauty through the transformative craft of semi-permanent eyebrows.

Our comprehensive program blends theory with hands-on practice, guiding aspiring artists through the intricacies of brow shaping, pigment selection, and advanced techniques in micro blading or shading.

Designed by industry experts, Andrea, Joanne and Anne Marie this course empowers individuals to master the delicate balance of art and technique, ensuring the creation of flawless, natural-looking brows while honing the skills necessary to thrive in the ever-evolving world of cosmetic enhancements. Join us and embark on a path that merges creativity with precision, sculpting confidence and artistry, one perfectly arched brow at a time

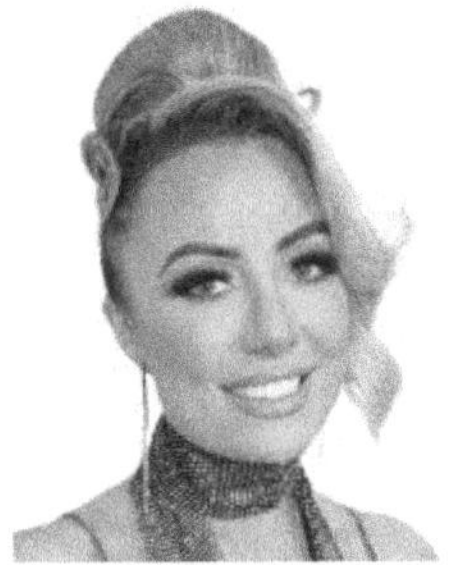

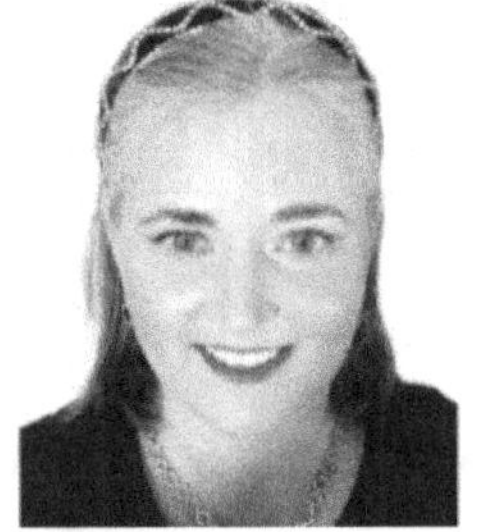

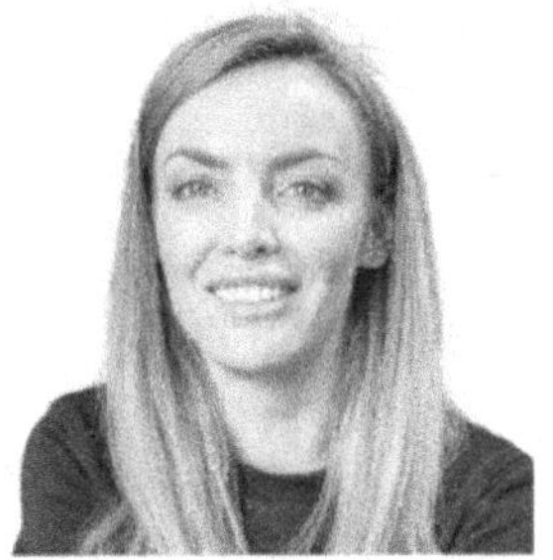

**Andrea Kirwin**

Andrea is an amazing beautician, an advanced skincare therapist, a semi-permanent make-up specialist, and a brow and lip expert

**Anne Marie McIlwraith**

Anne Marie is an experienced professional therapist, tutor, and entrepreneur

**Joanne Kelleher**

Joanne is an aesthetic skincare specialist and extension expert and barber

**Semi-Permanent Brow Training**

Course Title: Semi-Permanent Brow Training Course Duration: 5 Days (or as needed for comprehensive training)

**Lesson Plan for Semi-Permanent Brow Training**

### Day 1: Introduction to Semi-Permanent Brows

Overview of semi-permanent brow techniques (micro blading, micro shading, combination brows).

Understanding the benefits and applications of each technique.

Health and safety guidelines for brow procedures.

Discussion on skin anatomy relevant to brow procedures.

### Day 2: Brow Design and Mapping

Importance of brow design and symmetry.

Techniques for brow mapping based on face shape and client preferences.

Hands-on practice on brow mapping using live models.

### Day 3: Micro blading Technique

Introduction to micro blading tools and equipment.

Practice on artificial skin to master micro blading strokes.

Hands-on practice on live models under instructor supervision.

### Day 4: Micro shading Technique

Introduction to micro shading tools and equipment.

Techniques for creating soft, powder-like shading effects.

Practice on artificial skin and live models to perfect micro shading.

Understanding combination brows (micro blading + micro shading).

Practice on live models to create a gradient effect with crisp hair strokes and shading.

Discussion on touch-up procedures and aftercare instructions.

## Additional Topics (Optional):

Client Consultation and Consent Forms: Understanding the consultation process and obtaining informed consent from clients.

Colour Theory and Pigment Selection: Understanding pigment colour selection based on skin tone and client preferences.

Troubleshooting and Corrective Techniques: Strategies for addressing pigment retention issues and correcting uneven results.

Business and Marketing: Tips for setting up a semi-permanent brow business and marketing services effectively.

## Assessment and Certification:

Regular evaluations and feedback throughout the training program.

Final practical and written assessments to gauge proficiency in semi-permanent brow techniques.

Awarding of completion certificates to successful participants.

**Note:** The lesson plan can be adjusted based on the skill level of the trainees and the specific techniques being taught. The training is conducted by a qualified instructor with practical experience in semi-permanent brow procedures. Additionally, the instructor should emphasise the importance of ongoing practice and continued education for trainees to master their skills and maintain high-quality standards in their work.

**Training Program for Semi-Permanent Brow**
**(Micro blading/Micro shading)**

This training program for semi-permanent brows provides comprehensive education and hands-on experience to aspiring brow artists.

The program covers essential theoretical knowledge, practical skills, and safety protocols.
This is your training curriculum for semi-permanent brow techniques like micro blading and micro shading:

Semi-permanent brows can when professionally done, enhance the overall appearance of the client. It is essential that the client has confidence from their consultation with a trained and certified brow therapist before getting semi-permanent brows to discuss the best technique, expected results, and aftercare instructions.

Semi-permanent brows can be a game-changer for individuals looking to enhance their brows and streamline their beauty routines while enjoying natural-looking, long-lasting results

It's crucial for the brow therapist to communicate with the client to understand their preferences and expectations fully. By combining the client's preferences with a keen understanding of facial anatomy, a brow therapist can create a customised brow shape that enhances the client's beauty and complements their unique features.

In brow procedures, the therapist will be aware of the lymphatic drainage pathways to avoid excessive pigment migration. When performing semi-permanent brow procedures, the therapist will consider the depth of pigment implantation, as deeper penetration can lead to less crisp hair strokes and longer-lasting results, while shallower implantation may result in quicker fading.

It is important to understand the skin's healing process and ensure the client is informed particularly post-procedure care, as it is essential to ensure optimal pigment retention and satisfactory outcomes for the client. Comprehensive knowledge of the skin's layers and structures helps create safe, natural-looking, and long-lasting results while minimising potential risks and complications during the brow procedure

Certification in blood borne pathogen training is recommended to ensure understanding of infection prevention protocols.

By strictly following these health and safety guidelines, brow therapists can create a safe and clean environment for their clients and minimise the risk of infection or complications during and after the brow styling procedure.

The therapist will inquire about the client's medical history, including allergies and past reactions to cosmetics or procedures, and perform a patch test on a small area of the skin to check for pigment or anaesthetic allergies. It is important to assess the client's skin condition and overall health to determine if they are suitable candidates for the procedure. By taking allergies and contraindications into consideration and ensuring proper client assessment, brow therapists can minimise the risk of adverse reactions and provide a safe and successful brow styling experience for their clients. The professional will keep detailed records of the pigment mixtures used for each client, as this information will be valuable for touch-ups and future sessions.

The professional therapist will apply colour theory principles and carefully select pigments tailored to each client's skin tone; this will achieve natural and flattering results in semi-permanent brow styling. By mastering the art of pigment mixing, brow therapists can provide customised and natural-looking semi-permanent brow results that enhance their clients' facial features and complement their unique appearances.

By mastering the art of pigment correction and adjustment, a brow therapist can address any colour-related challenges that may arise during the semi-permanent brow styling process, leading to natural-looking and flattering results that enhance the client's overall appearance.
Using high-quality and sterile tools and equipment are essential to ensure the safety and success of semi-permanent brow procedures. Proper maintenance and adherence to hygiene standards are crucial for the well-being of both the brow therapist and the client

Understanding the various needle configurations and their applications allows brow therapists to select the most suitable technique for each client and create customised, natural-looking, and flattering results. It's important for therapists to have proper training and experience in using different needles to ensure safe and successful semi-permanent brow procedures

By effectively managing client expectations and providing clear and thorough aftercare instructions, brow therapists can ensure that their clients have a positive and rewarding semi-permanent brow experience, leading to beautiful and long-lasting results

Conducting a patch test is a crucial safety measure to identify and avoid potential allergic reactions. Brow therapists should never skip this step, and they should take any client-reported reactions seriously, adjusting the pigments or products as needed to ensure the client's safety and well-being during the semi-permanent brow procedure.

By using correct brow mapping techniques, brow therapists can create balanced and symmetrical brows that enhance the client's facial features and complement their overall appearance. Regular practice and attention to detail are key to mastering this essential aspect of semi-permanent brow procedures. Paying attention to facial proportions and customising the brow shape to suit the client's features will lead to satisfying and flattering results in semi-permanent brow procedures.

Regular touch-up sessions are essential for maintaining the semi-permanent brows' appearance and ensuring long-lasting, beautiful results. By identifying the need for touch-ups and performing them with precision and care, you can help your clients maintain their desired brow look and ensure their satisfaction with the semi-permanent brow procedure

## Module 1: Introduction to Semi-Permanent Brows

Semi-Permanent Brows:      Understanding the concept of semi-permanent brows and their benefits.

### Understanding Semi-Permanent Brows:

Semi-permanent brows refer to a set of cosmetic procedures designed to enhance and improve the appearance of eyebrows in a semi-permanent manner. Unlike traditional eyebrow makeup, such as eyebrow pencils or powders, semi-permanent brows involve implanting pigments into the skin to create natural-looking results that can last for an extended period, typically between 12 to 24 months. The two most common techniques used for semi-permanent brows are micro blading and micro shading.

### Benefits of Semi-Permanent Brows:

**Enhanced Appearance:** Semi-permanent brows can significantly enhance the appearance of eyebrows, creating a more defined and polished look. They can add fullness, shape, and symmetry to sparse or uneven brows, resulting in a more aesthetically pleasing facial appearance.

**Natural-Looking Results:** When performed by a skilled and experienced brow artist, semi-permanent brow techniques like micro blading and micro shading can produce results that closely resemble natural eyebrow hairs. This natural-looking effect is achieved through meticulous brow mapping and precise application techniques.

**Time-Saving:** One of the main benefits of semi-permanent brows is the time saved on daily eyebrow grooming. Clients no longer need to spend time filling in their eyebrows with makeup products each day, as the semi-permanent pigments maintain the desired brow shape and fullness.

**Long-Lasting Results:** While semi-permanent brows are not permanent tattoos, they do have significantly longer staying power compared to traditional makeup. Depending on the technique used and individual factors, the results can last anywhere from 12 to 24 months, reducing the need for frequent touch-ups.

**Customisation:** Semi-permanent brow procedures can be tailored to suit each client's unique facial features, skin tone, and desired brow shape. This customisation ensures that the final results complement the client's overall appearance.

**Confidence Boost:** For individuals with thin or sparse eyebrows, semi-permanent brows can provide a confidence boost by restoring or enhancing their natural eyebrow appearance. Well-defined brows frame the face and can make a significant difference in one's overall self-esteem.

**Semi-Reversible:** Unlike permanent tattoos, semi-permanent brow techniques allow for some flexibility in making changes or adjustments over time. As the pigments gradually fade, clients can opt for different shapes or colours during subsequent touch-up sessions.

**Minimal Downtime:** Semi-permanent brow procedures typically involve minimal downtime, and clients can resume their regular activities shortly after the treatment.

- 

<table>
<tr><td>Semi-Permanent Brows:</td><td>Overview of micro blading and micro shading techniques.</td></tr>
</table>

**Overview of Micro blading and Micro shading Techniques for Brows**

Micro blading and micro shading are semi-permanent brow enhancement techniques that have gained popularity for their ability to create natural-looking, well-defined eyebrows. These procedures are typically performed by trained professionals known as brow artists or micro blading technicians. Let's explore the key features of each technique:

**Micro blading:**

Micro blading is a manual method of implanting pigment into the skin to create hair stroke-like lines that mimic natural eyebrow hairs.

A handheld tool with a cluster of fine needles, called a micro blade, is used to make small, precise incisions in the epidermal layer of the skin.

Pigment is then deposited into these tiny incisions, resulting in individual, crisp hair strokes that blend seamlessly with existing eyebrow hairs. Micro blading is ideal for clients with thin or sparse eyebrows, as it adds fullness and definition to the brows.

The technique requires meticulous brow mapping and careful attention to detail to achieve symmetrical and balanced results. Micro bladed brows can last from 12 to 18 months, depending on the client's skin type, lifestyle, and aftercare.

**Micro shading:**

Micro shading is a semi-permanent brow technique that involves creating a soft, powdered effect on the eyebrows, similar to the look achieved with eyebrow powder or pencil.

Instead of hair strokes, micro shading uses a stippling method with a manual tool or a tattoo machine to create small, controlled dots of pigment.

This technique is well-suited for clients with thicker natural eyebrows who desire a more defined and filled-in appearance.

Micro shading can also be combined with micro blading (referred to as a combination or ombré brow) to achieve a gradient effect, with a defined tail and softly shaded front.

The results of micro shading are softer and more diffused compared to micro blading.

Micro shaded brows can last from 12 to 24 months, depending on individual factors and proper aftercare.

Combination brows involve a combination of micro blading and micro shading techniques to achieve a textured, multidimensional look.

This approach is particularly useful for clients with minimal natural brow hair who desire a fuller, yet natural-looking result.

The hair strokes created with micro blading add a realistic look to the brow, while the shading technique provides density and definition.

Combination brows can last from 12 to 24 months, depending on skin type, pigment retention, and aftercare.

Both micro blading and micro shading require meticulous brow design, precise technique, and adherence to strict health and safety standards. Clients should be provided with detailed aftercare instructions to ensure proper healing and colour retention.
It's important to consult with a trained and experienced brow artist before choosing a technique to determine which one best suits your natural brow type and desired look.

<table>
<tr><td>Semi-Permanent Brows:</td><td>Different brow styles and shapes based on face anatomy and client preferences.</td></tr>
</table>

Brows come in various styles and shapes, and choosing the right one depends on the client's facial anatomy and personal preferences. A skilled brow artist considers the client's unique features and desired look to create a well-balanced and flattering brow shape. Here are some popular brow styles based on different face shapes and client preferences:

**1. Classic Arched Brows:**
Suitable for most face shapes.
Features a defined arch that starts near the centre of the brow and gradually tapers towards the tail.
Provides a lifted appearance and a more expressive look.

**2. Soft Arched Brows:**
Ideal for clients with more delicate facial features.
Similar to classic arched brows but with a gentler and less pronounced arch.
Creates a subtle, natural-looking lift to the eyes.

**3. Straight Brows:**
Works well for clients with round or square face shapes.
Features a horizontal brow shape without a pronounced arch.
Gives a youthful, soft, and balanced appearance to the face.

**4. S-Shaped Brows:**
A modern and trendy brow style.
Starts with a soft arch near the centre of the brow, then curves downwards, and finally lifts slightly at the tail.
Suits clients with oval or heart-shaped faces.

**5. Rounded Brows:**
Suitable for clients with angular face shapes (e.g., square or diamond).
Features a soft curve with no defined arch, creating a more rounded appearance.
Adds softness and femininity to the face.

**6. Feathered Brows:**
A popular choice for clients with sparse or thin brows.
Involves creating soft, feathery strokes to mimic natural brow hairs.
Provides a fuller and more textured appearance.

**7. Bold Brows:**
Ideal for clients with strong facial features and a bold personality.
Features a thicker and more prominent brow shape with a defined arch.
Adds intensity and character to the face.

**8. Short Brows:**
Suitable for clients with longer faces or high foreheads.
Involves creating a shorter brow shape to balance the proportions of the face.
Provides a more proportionate and harmonious appearance.

**9. Long Brows:**
Works well for clients with round or square faces.
Involves extending the length of the brows slightly to elongate the face.
Creates a more elegant and elongated look.

**10. Natural Brows:**
Suitable for clients who prefer a minimalistic and effortless look.
Enhances the client's natural brow shape with subtle grooming and colouring.
Emphasises the client's individuality and features.

**Module 2: Skin Anatomy and Safety Protocols**
Semi-Permanent Brows:       Study of skin layers and structures relevant to brow procedures.

Studying the skin layers and structures relevant to brow procedures is essential for brow artists to perform safe and effective semi-permanent brow techniques like micro blading and micro shading.

Understanding the skin's anatomy ensures that the pigments are deposited at the appropriate depth and that the procedures are well-tolerated by the clients. Here's an overview of the skin layers and structures relevant to brow procedures:

**1. Epidermis:**
The epidermis is the outermost layer of the skin.

It is composed of several sublayers, including the stratum corneum (the most superficial layer) and the basal layer (the innermost layer).  In brow procedures, the pigment is deposited into the epidermis to create hair strokes or shading effects.

**2. Dermis:**
The dermis lies beneath the epidermis and is a thicker layer of connective tissue.

It contains blood vessels, nerves, hair follicles, and sebaceous glands.

The dermis plays a vital role in the skin's structural integrity and nutrient supply.

**3. Hair Follicles:**
Hair follicles are tiny structures within the dermis that produce hair.

In brow procedures, hair follicles may be a reference point for creating hair strokes that mimic natural eyebrow hairs.

**4. Sebaceous Glands:**
Sebaceous glands produce sebum, which is an oily substance that lubricates and protects the skin.

The presence of sebaceous glands can influence how pigments are retained in the skin.

**5. Capillaries and Blood Vessels:**
Capillaries and blood vessels supply oxygen and nutrients to the skin cells.

During the brow procedure, some bleeding may occur due to the penetration of blood vessels.

This is important for the artist to consider when selecting the depth of pigment insertion.

## 6. Nerve Endings:
The skin contains nerve endings that are responsible for the sense of touch and pain perception.

Understanding the location of nerve endings is crucial to ensure the client's comfort during the procedure.

## 7. Lymphatic System:
The lymphatic system plays a role in the body's immune response and waste removal.

<table><tr><td>Semi-Permanent Brows:</td><td>Health and safety guidelines, including infection control and sanitation procedures.</td></tr></table>

Brow styling, particularly semi-permanent brow procedures like micro blading and micro shading, requires strict adherence to health and safety guidelines to ensure the well-being of both the clients and the brow artists. Infection control and sanitation procedures are critical to prevent the transmission of pathogens and maintain a clean and hygienic environment. Here are some key health and safety guidelines for brow styling:

**1. Personal Protective Equipment (PPE):**
Brow artists should wear disposable gloves, face masks, and other appropriate PPE during the entire procedure.

Gloves should be changed between clients to prevent cross-contamination.

**2. Hand Hygiene:**
Brow artists should thoroughly wash their hands with soap and water before and after each client.

Hand sanitisers with at least 60% alcohol content can be used in addition to handwashing.

**3. Sterilisation and Disinfection:**
All tools and equipment used during the procedure, such as micro blading pens, blades, and shading needles, must be properly sterilised before use.

Non-disposable tools should be cleaned and disinfected with an appropriate solution between clients.

Disposable tools and single-use items should be discarded properly after each use.

**4. Surface Disinfection:**
All workstations, treatment beds, and surfaces in the treatment area should be thoroughly cleaned and disinfected before and after each client.

Disinfectants with proven efficacy against bacteria, viruses, and blood borne pathogens should be used.

**5. Client Health Assessment:**
Prior to the procedure, clients should be screened for any signs of illness, recent infections, or skin conditions that may contraindicate the treatment.

Clients with contagious conditions or compromised immune systems should not be treated until they have recovered.

### 6. Disposable Barriers:

Disposable barrier films or covers should be used to protect treatment beds and other equipment from contamination and facilitate easy clean-up.

### 7. Waste Disposal:

All disposable items, such as gloves, cotton pads, and tissues, used during the procedure should be disposed of in sealed, designated waste containers.

### 8. Pre-Procedure Preparation:

Brow artists should thoroughly clean and disinfect their hands and work area before beginning the procedure.

Clients' brows and surrounding skin should be cleansed with an appropriate antiseptic solution before starting the treatment.

### 9. Aftercare Instructions:

Clients should be provided with detailed aftercare instructions to minimise the risk of infection and promote proper healing.

Emphasise the importance of avoiding touching the treated area and keeping it clean and dry during the healing process.

### 10. Regular Training and Certification:

Brow artists should undergo regular training on infection control and sanitation procedures to stay updated on best practices.

Brow styling, especially semi-permanent brow procedures like micro blading and micro shading, requires careful consideration of potential allergies and contraindications that may affect the procedure's safety and success. Identifying and addressing these factors is essential to ensure the well-being of the clients and to avoid adverse reactions. Here are common allergies and contraindications to be aware of:

**Allergies:**
**Pigment Allergy:** Some individuals may be allergic to the pigments used in semi-permanent brow procedures. This can result in itching, redness, swelling, or other allergic reactions on the treated area.

**Topical Aesthetic Allergy:** Brow artists often use topical anaesthetics to numb the area before the procedure. Clients may have allergies to certain anaesthetic ingredients, which could cause skin irritation or an allergic reaction.

**Latex Allergy:** Some disposable gloves and other materials used during the procedure may contain latex, which can trigger allergic reactions in clients with latex allergies.

**Contraindications:**
**Pregnancy and Breastfeeding:** Performing semi-permanent brow procedures on pregnant or breastfeeding clients is generally not recommended due to hormonal changes and the potential impact on pigment retention and healing.

**Skin Conditions:** Clients with skin conditions like eczema, psoriasis, active acne, or open wounds on the brow area should avoid the procedure until the condition has cleared up.

**History of Keloids or Hypertrophic Scarring:** Clients with a history of keloid or hypertrophic scarring may be at a higher risk of developing excessive scarring in the treated area.

**Blood Disorders and Medications:** Certain blood disorders or medications that affect blood clotting may increase the risk of bleeding during the procedure.

**Recent Botox or Fillers:** Clients who have received Botox or dermal fillers in the brow area should wait at least two weeks before undergoing a brow styling procedure.

**History of Allergic Reactions to Tattoos or Permanent Makeup:** Clients who have experienced allergic reactions to previous tattoos or permanent makeup procedures may not be suitable candidates for semi-permanent brow styling.

**Client Consultation:** Conducting a thorough client consultation is crucial to identify any allergies or contraindications that may affect the procedure. During the consultation, the brow artist should:

**Module 3: Colour Theory and Pigment Selection**

Semi-Permanent Brows:     Colour theory principles and how to choose pigments suitable for different skin tones.

Colour theory principles play a crucial role in semi-permanent brow styling, as choosing the right pigments that complement different skin tones can significantly impact the final results. Understanding colour theory helps brow artists achieve natural-looking and harmonious outcomes for their clients. Here are the key colour theory principles and guidelines for selecting pigments suitable for different skin tones:

**1. Undertones:**
Undertones refer to the subtle hues beneath the surface of the skin. They can be categorised as warm, cool, or neutral.

Warm undertones: Skin with yellow, peach, or golden undertones.

Cool undertones: Skin with pink, red, or blue undertones.

Neutral undertones: Skin with a balanced mix of warm and cool tones.

**2. Complementary Colours:**
Complementary colours are pairs of colours that are located opposite each other on the colour wheel.

For warm undertones (e.g., yellow), complementary pigments with cool undertones (e.g., ashy brown) can create a balanced and natural appearance.

For cool undertones (e.g., pink), complementary pigments with warm undertones (e.g., golden brown) can provide a harmonious effect.

**3. Choosing Pigments for Different Skin Tones:**
Fair Skin: Clients with fair skin often have lighter hair colours. Light to medium ash or cool brown pigments can work well to achieve a soft and natural look. Avoid using pigments that are too dark or warm, as they may look unnatural on fair skin.

Medium Skin: For clients with medium skin tones, a range of warm and cool brown pigments can be suitable, depending on their natural hair colour. Medium brown or taupe shades often work best for medium skin tones.

Olive Skin: Olive skin tones can vary in undertones. Brown pigments with slightly warmer or neutral tones tend to blend well with olive skin and complement the natural brow colour.

Dark Skin: For clients with dark skin tones, using dark brown or black pigments can provide definition and intensity. Care should be taken not to go too dark, as it may create a harsh contrast.

## 4. Patch Tests:

Before the actual procedure, it is essential to perform patch tests on a small area of the skin to check for pigment allergies and ensure the chosen colour blends well with the client's skin tone.

## 5. Customisation and Mixing:

Brow artists should be skilled in customising pigments to suit individual clients. Mixing different pigment shades allows for more precise colour matching.

## 6. Client Consultation:

During the consultation, engage in a conversation with the client to understand their preferences and desired outcomes.

Assess the client's natural hair colour and skin undertones to make informed pigment selections.

In semi-permanent brow styling, mixing pigments is a skill that allows brow artists to achieve the desired shades and undertones that best complement the client's natural hair colour and skin tone. Customising pigments ensures that the results appear natural and harmonious with the client's overall appearance. Here are some essential tips for mixing pigments effectively:

**1. Understanding Pigment Colours:**
Familiarise yourself with the primary pigment colours commonly used in brow styling, such as brown, black, blonde, taupe, and ashy tones.

Different pigment manufacturers may have varying colour charts, so it's essential to be familiar with the specific pigments you work with.

**2. Assessing Client's Natural Hair Colour and Skin Tone:**
Before starting the procedure, carefully assess the client's natural hair colour and skin tone to determine the appropriate pigment shades and undertones.

Consider the client's undertones (warm, cool, or neutral) and adjust the pigment mixture accordingly to achieve a harmonious match.

**3. Start with Small Amounts:**
When mixing pigments, start with small amounts of each colour to avoid wasting pigments or creating an overly saturated mixture.

It's easier to add more pigment to the mixture than to dilute it if it becomes too intense.

**4. Mixing Techniques:**
Use a clean and disposable pigment cup or mixing ring to prevent cross-contamination.

Use a micro brush or dropper to add small drops of pigments to the cup.

Gradually mix the pigments together using a micro brush or a sterile mixing stick until you achieve the desired shade.

**5. Trial and Error:**
Pigment mixing may require some trial and error, especially when working with new clients or unique skin tones.

Keep a record of the pigment mixtures used for each client to refer back to for future touch-ups or adjustments.

**6. Test the Mixture:**

Before applying the mixed pigment to the client's brows, perform a patch test on a small area of the skin to check for allergies and to ensure that the colour matches the client's expectations.

## 7. Customisation for Each Brow:
Remember that eyebrows are not always symmetrical, and the shade may differ slightly between the two brows.

Adjust the pigment mixture slightly for each brow to achieve a natural and balanced result.

## 8. Seek Advanced Training:
To become proficient in pigment mixing and achieve consistent and exceptional results, consider seeking advanced training and continuing education in semi-permanent brow styling.

## 9. Documentation:
Keep detailed records of the pigment mixtures used for each client, as this information will be valuable for touch-ups and future sessions.

<table>
<tr><td>Semi-Permanent Brows:</td><td>Correcting and adjusting pigment colours for natural-looking results.</td></tr>
</table>

Correcting and adjusting pigment colours is a crucial skill in semi-permanent brow styling to achieve natural-looking results and address any pigment-related issues that may arise during or after the procedure. Whether the colour needs to be softened, darkened, or corrected, a brow artist must be skilled in making precise adjustments. Here are some techniques for correcting and adjusting pigment colours:

**1. Colour Neutralisers:**
Colour neutralisers are used to counteract unwanted undertones in the pigment.

For example, if the pigment appears too warm or red-toned on the skin, a green or cool-toned colour neutraliser can help balance it out.

**2. Colour Balancing:**
Brow artists can adjust the pigment colour by adding small amounts of complementary pigments to achieve the desired shade.

For instance, if the pigment is too warm, adding a touch of a cooler colour can balance the warmth and create a more natural look.

**3. Lightening and Darkening:**
Lightening or darkening pigments is achieved by adding a lighter or darker shade to the existing pigment.
Gradual adjustments should be made to avoid drastic changes and to ensure a smooth transition between colours.

**4. Pigment Removal:**
In some cases, when a pigment colour is too intense or undesirable, a pigment removal solution can be used to lighten the colour.

Pigment removal should be performed with caution to avoid causing damage to the skin.

**5. Patch Tests:**
Before making any significant pigment adjustments on a client's brows, perform patch tests on a small area of the skin to check for allergic reactions or adverse effects.

**6. Gradual Corrections:**
When correcting pigment colours, it's essential to make gradual adjustments rather than attempting to fix the issue all at once.

Multiple sessions may be required to achieve the desired results, especially if the client's skin takes longer to heal or retain pigment.

**7. Avoiding Overcorrection:**
Brow artists should be cautious not to overcorrect the pigment colour, as this can lead to unnatural-looking results.

Continuously reassess the client's brows throughout the healing process to determine if additional adjustments are necessary.

**8. Experience and Skill:**
Correcting and adjusting pigment colours require experience, skill, and a keen eye for colour.

Brow artists should seek advanced training and hands-on practice to become proficient in pigment corrections.

**9. Transparent Communication:**
Be transparent and communicative with the client about the need for adjustments and the expected outcome.

Managing client expectations is crucial to ensure satisfaction with the final results.

**Module 4: Tools and Equipment**

<table>
<tr><td>Semi-Permanent Brows:</td><td>Overview of the tools and equipment used in semi-permanent brow procedures.</td></tr>
</table>

In semi-permanent brow styling, various tools and equipment are used to perform procedures like micro blading, micro shading, and combination brows. These tools are essential for achieving precise and natural-looking results. Here are the common tools and equipment used in semi-permanent brow procedures:

**1. Micro blading Pen or Hand Tool:**
A micro blading pen or hand tool is used to create fine, precise hair strokes in the brow area.

The tool holds a cluster of ultra-fine needles that allow for controlled pigment implantation.

**2. Micro blades:**
Micro blades come in various configurations, such as U-shaped, curved, or straight needles.

They are disposable and should be single-use to maintain hygiene and prevent cross-contamination.

**3. Micro shading or Shading Tools:**
For micro shading or ombre brow techniques, different shading tools are used to create soft, powder-like effects.

These tools may include shading pens, manual shading blades, or shading needles.

**4. Pigments:**
Semi-permanent brow pigments are formulated specifically for cosmetic tattooing.

They come in a range of colours to match different brow hair shades and skin tones.

**5. Topical Anaesthetics:**
Topical anaesthetics are used to numb the brow area and minimise discomfort during the procedure.
They are typically applied before the micro blading or micro shading process.

**6. Pigment Cups and Rings:**
Disposable pigment cups or rings are used to hold and mix pigments.

They allow for easy access to pigments during the procedure.

**7. Pigment Rings:**
Pigment rings are small, disposable rings that are worn on the finger, making it convenient for the artist to dip the micro blade or shading tool into the pigment.

**8. Micro brushes or Cotton Swabs:**

Micro brushes or cotton swabs are used to apply anaesthetic, remove excess pigment, and clean the brow area during the procedure.

**9. Rulers and Callipers:**
Rulers and callipers are used to measure and mark the brow shape accurately during the brow mapping process.

**10. Barrier Films and Covers:**
Barrier films or covers are used to protect equipment and work surfaces from contamination.

They provide a barrier against bacteria and help maintain a clean environment.

**11. Aftercare Products:**
Aftercare products, such as post-procedure creams or ointments, are provided to clients to promote proper healing and colour retention.

**12. Disposable Gloves:**
Disposable gloves are worn by the brow artist to maintain a sterile and hygienic environment.

Gloves should be changed between clients to avoid cross-contamination.

**13. Alcohol Wipes and Antiseptic Solutions:**
Alcohol wipes and antiseptic solutions are used for disinfection and preparation of the brow area before the procedure.

Proper handling and care of needles, hand tools, and machines are crucial for ensuring the safety and hygiene of semi-permanent brow procedures. Here are important guidelines to follow:

**1. Sterilisation and Disinfection:**
Before each procedure, sterilise all reusable tools, such as needles, hand tools, and machine parts, using an autoclave or an approved Sterilisation method.

Disinfect all non-sterilisable items with an appropriate high-level disinfectant between each client.

**2. Single-Use Policy:**
Use single-use, disposable needles for each client to prevent cross-contamination.

Dispose of used needles and other single-use items in a sharps container immediately after the procedure.

**3. Glove Usage:**
Wear disposable, latex-free gloves during each procedure to protect yourself and your clients from potential infections.

Change gloves between clients and whenever there is a risk of contamination.

**4. Sanitisation of Work Area:**
Thoroughly clean and sanitise your work area before and after each client.
Use disposable barrier films or plastic wraps to cover work surfaces and equipment for easy clean-up.

**5. Hand Washing:**
Wash your hands with soap and water for at least 20 seconds before and after each procedure.
Use hand sanitiser with at least 60% alcohol if hand washing facilities are not available.

**6. Handling Needles and Tools:**
Handle needles, hand tools, and machine parts with care to avoid damage or contamination.

Avoid touching the needle's sharp tip, and use a needle holder or tweezers for safe handling.

**7. Needle Disposal:**
Dispose of used needles properly in a sharps container according to local regulations.

Secure the sharps container and arrange for appropriate disposal when it is full.

**8. Maintenance of Hand Tools and Machines:**

Regularly inspect and clean hand tools and machines to ensure proper functioning and hygiene.

Follow the manufacturer's instructions for maintenance and cleaning.

**9. Protective Barriers:**
Use disposable, single-use barriers on machines and hand tools to prevent direct contact with the client's skin.

Change these barriers between clients to maintain cleanliness.

**10. Training and Education:**
Stay up-to-date with industry best practices and attend training courses to enhance your knowledge of proper needle handling and hygiene.

Regularly refresh your knowledge of safety protocols and sanitation procedures.

In semi-permanent brow procedures, different needle configurations are used to achieve various effects and hair strokes. Understanding the different needle configurations and their applications is essential for brow artists to create natural-looking and customised results for their clients. Here are some common needle configurations and their applications:

**1. Single Needle (Round):**
The single needle, also known as a round needle, is a basic and versatile needle configuration.

It is used for creating thin, fine, and precise hair strokes in micro blading.

Ideal for clients with thin or sparse brows, as it mimics the appearance of natural eyebrow hairs.

**2. Slanted Needle (Flat):

The slanted needle, also known as a flat needle, has a flat configuration with a slanted edge.

It is used for shading and soft ombre effects in micro shading techniques.
The slanted shape allows for smoother and more even pigment distribution, resulting in a powder-like finish.

**3. U-Shape Needle (Curved):
The U-shape needle, also known as a curved needle, has a rounded configuration with a slight curve.

It is used for creating soft, natural-looking hair strokes with a gentle arch.

Suitable for clients who desire a more subtle and delicate brow appearance.

**4. Double Row Needle:
The double row needle consists of two rows of fine needles arranged closely together.

It is used for creating denser and fuller hair strokes, especially for clients with sparse or missing brow hair.

Provides a quicker and more efficient procedure for adding volume to the brows.

**5. Blade and Shader Combination:
Some needle configurations combine a blade (for hair strokes) with a shading component (for powder or soft shading effects).

This combination is used for combination brows, where hair strokes are incorporated with shading to achieve a more defined and textured look.

**6. Fine and Thick Needles:

Needles come in varying thicknesses (gauges), ranging from extra fine to thick.

Fine needles are used for delicate hair strokes and more precise work, while thicker needles are used for denser shading or bold hair strokes.

**7. Needle Groupings:
Needle groupings refer to the arrangement of multiple needles together in a single configuration.

Common needle groupings include 3, 5, 7, or more needles.

Different groupings are used based on the desired effect and the density required.

**8. Micro blade and Micro shading Needles:
Micro blading needles typically have a single or a few fine needles for hair strokes.

Micro shading needles usually have a row or cluster of needles for shading effects.

## Module 5: Pre-Procedure Preparation

<table>
<tr><td>Semi-Permanent Brows:</td><td>Consultation techniques to understand client expectations and preferences.</td></tr>
</table>

Conducting a thorough consultation is a crucial step in the semi-permanent brow process. Proper consultation techniques allow brow artists to understand their client's expectations, preferences, and individual needs. Here are some effective consultation techniques to ensure a successful and satisfying semi-permanent brow experience:

**1. Active Listening:**
Begin the consultation by actively listening to the client's desires and concerns.

Allow the client to express their preferences and expectations openly without interruption.

**2. Client Questionnaire:**
Use a client questionnaire to gather essential information about the client's medical history, past cosmetic procedures, allergies, and current medications.

Include questions about their brow preferences, desired shape, colour, and any specific concerns.

**3. Assess Natural Brows:**
Observe the client's natural brows to understand their current shape, thickness, and any potential issues.

Ask the client about their feelings towards their natural brows and what specific changes they'd like to see.

**4. Brow Mapping:**
Use brow mapping techniques to demonstrate potential brow shapes and designs.
Involve the client in the mapping process to ensure their preferences are considered.

**5. Show Before and After Pictures:**
Show the client before and after pictures of previous work you have done to manage their expectations.

Ensure the examples are of clients with similar facial features and skin tones.

**6. Communicate the Process:**
Explain the semi-permanent brow process in detail, including the procedure steps, healing time, and expected results.

Discuss any potential risks or complications.

**7. Colour Selection:**
Determine the client's natural hair colour and skin tone to choose pigments that best suit them.

Show different pigment options to the client and explain how colour selection can enhance their features.

**8. Set Realistic Expectations:**
Be honest with the client about what can be achieved with semi-permanent brows, considering their natural brow shape and hair growth patterns.

Educate the client on the healing process and that the final results will be apparent after the brows have healed.

**9. Client Feedback and Consent:**
Encourage the client to ask questions and provide feedback during the consultation.

Obtain informed consent for the procedure, ensuring the client is fully aware of the potential outcomes and aftercare requirements.

**10. Offer Customisation:**
Tailor the semi-permanent brow procedure to the client's preferences and facial features.

Consider their lifestyle and daily makeup routine when suggesting brow styles.

Managing client expectations and providing comprehensive aftercare instructions are essential aspects of ensuring a successful and satisfactory semi-permanent brow experience. Properly managing expectations and offering clear aftercare guidance help clients understand the healing process and contribute to long-lasting and beautiful results. Here are some key tips for managing client expectations and providing aftercare instructions:

## 1. Clear Communication:

During the consultation and before the procedure, communicate openly and honestly with the client about the expected outcomes.

Be realistic about the results and the healing process.

## 2. Educate on the Healing Process:

Explain to the client that the brows will appear darker and more intense immediately after the procedure.

Inform them that the colour will soften and settle during the healing process.

## 3. Duration of Healing:

Let the client know that the complete healing process typically takes around 4 to 6 weeks.

Explain that the final results will be evident after the skin has fully healed.

## 4. Individual Variations:

Emphasise that every individual heals differently, and the retention of pigment can vary from person to person.

Results may depend on factors such as skin type, lifestyle, and aftercare adherence.

## 5. Possible Touch-Ups:

Inform the client that a touch-up session may be necessary to perfect the brows and achieve the desired results.

Explain the importance of attending the touch-up appointment, usually scheduled 4 to 8 weeks after the initial procedure.

## 6. Aftercare Instructions:

Provide the client with detailed aftercare instructions in writing and verbally.

Explain the importance of following the aftercare guidelines to ensure proper healing and colour retention.

**7. Avoiding Certain Activities:**
Advise the client to avoid activities that may compromise the healing process, such as excessive sweating, swimming, or exposure to direct sunlight.

**8. No Picking or Scratching:**
Stress the importance of not picking or scratching the treated area during the healing process, as this can lead to pigment loss.

**9. Use of Aftercare Products:**
Recommend the use of aftercare products, such as healing creams or ointments, to promote a smooth healing process.

**10. Schedule Follow-Up Appointments:**
Schedule follow-up appointments to check on the healing progress and address any concerns the client may have.

**11. Support:**
Let the client know that they can reach out to you with any questions or concerns they may have during the healing process.

Conducting patch tests is a crucial step in the semi-permanent brow process to identify potential allergic reactions to pigments or other products used during the procedure. Patch tests help ensure the safety and well-being of clients, especially those who may have sensitive skin or a history of allergies. Here's how to conduct a patch test for potential allergic reactions:

**1. Explanation and Consent:**
Before the consultation or the day of the procedure, explain to the client the purpose and importance of the patch test.

Obtain the client's consent to perform the test, ensuring they understand its significance in ensuring their safety.

**2. Selecting the Test Area:**
Choose a small and inconspicuous area on the client's forearm or behind the ear for the patch test.

Make sure the area is clean and free from any skin irritations or open wounds.

**3. Preparing the Test Materials:**
Prepare a small amount of the pigment that will be used during the semi-permanent brow procedure.

Mix it according to the manufacturer's instructions and use a sterile micro brush to apply the pigment to the test area.

**4. Patch Test Application:**
Apply a small amount of the pigment to the test area using the micro brush.

Ensure the pigment is not mixed with any anaesthetics or other products during the patch test.

**5. Record Keeping:**
Take note of the pigment used, the date and time of the patch test, and any observations made during and after the application.

**6. Monitoring the Test Area:**
Instruct the client to leave the patch test area untouched for at least 48 hours.

Advise them to avoid excessive water contact or exposure to direct sunlight during this period.

**7. Observations and Reactions:**

Instruct the client to monitor the test area for any signs of redness, itching, swelling, or other allergic reactions.

Encourage them to report any discomfort or abnormal reactions to you during the 48-hour monitoring period.

**8. Interpretation of Results:**
After 48 hours, examine the test area to check for any adverse reactions.

If the client experiences an allergic reaction, refrain from proceeding with the semi-permanent brow procedure, and recommend they seek medical advice.

**9. Documenting the Results:**
Record the results of the patch test in the client's file for future reference.

If the client passes the patch test without any adverse reactions, you can proceed with the scheduled semi-permanent brow procedure.

## Module 6: Brow Design and Mapping

| Semi-Permanent Brows: | Correct brow mapping techniques for balanced and symmetrical brows. |
| --- | --- |

Correct brow mapping techniques are essential for achieving balanced and symmetrical brows in semi-permanent brow procedures. Proper brow mapping ensures that the brows are tailored to the client's unique facial features and proportions, resulting in natural-looking and flattering results. Here are the steps for correct brow mapping techniques:

**1. Identify Key Facial Reference Points:**
Begin by identifying key facial reference points, such as the inner corner (starting point), arch, and outer corner (end point) of each eyebrow.

Use these points as the foundation for creating balanced and symmetrical brows.

**2. Measure the Brow Starting Point:**
Use a straight object, such as a ruler or brow mapping tool, to measure the distance from the centre of the nostril to the starting point of each brow.

Mark this point lightly with a brow pencil or a removable marking pen.

**3. Find the Brow Arch Position:**
Align the straight object diagonally from the centre of the nostril to the outer edge of the iris (the coloured part of the eye) to determine the arch position.

Mark this point lightly with the brow pencil.

**4. Determine the Brow End Point:**
Place the straight object diagonally from the centre of the nostril to the outer corner of the eye to determine the end point of the brow.

Mark this point lightly with the brow pencil.

**5. Create the Tail of the Brow:**
To ensure a natural and gradual brow taper, place the straight object diagonally from the arch point to the end point.

Mark this point lightly with the brow pencil to create the tail of the brow.

**6. Double-Check Symmetry:**
Compare the markings of both brows to ensure they are symmetrical and balanced.

Adjust the markings as needed to achieve harmony between the two brows.

**7. Adjust Brow Thickness and Shape:**
Take into consideration the client's facial structure, eye shape, and personal preferences when determining the ideal brow thickness and shape.

Use the brow mapping as a guide to create a shape that complements the client's features.

**8. Finalise the Brow Design:**
Once the brow mapping is complete and both brows are symmetrical, finalise the brow design with the client's approval.

Discuss the proposed shape and make any adjustments based on the client's feedback.

**9. Hair Growth Patterns:**
Consider the client's natural hair growth patterns when creating hair strokes or shading to ensure a realistic and natural appearance.

**10. Brow Mapping Tools:**
Brow mapping tools, such as rulers with various measurements, can aid in achieving precise and balanced brow mapping.

Some artists may also use thread or specialised callipers for accuracy.

Correct brow mapping techniques are essential for achieving balanced and symmetrical brows in semi-permanent brow procedures. Proper brow mapping ensures that the brows are tailored to the client's unique facial features and proportions, resulting in natural-looking and flattering results. Here are the steps for correct brow mapping techniques:

**1. Identify Key Facial Reference Points:**
Begin by identifying key facial reference points, such as the inner corner (starting point), arch, and outer corner (end point) of each eyebrow.

Use these points as the foundation for creating balanced and symmetrical brows.

**2. Measure the Brow Starting Point:**
Use a straight object, such as a ruler or brow mapping tool, to measure the distance from the centre of the nostril to the starting point of each brow.

Mark this point lightly with a brow pencil or a removable marking pen.

**3. Find the Brow Arch Position:**
Align the straight object diagonally from the centre of the nostril to the outer edge of the iris (the coloured part of the eye) to determine the arch position.

Mark this point lightly with the brow pencil.

**4. Determine the Brow End Point:**
Place the straight object diagonally from the centre of the nostril to the outer corner of the eye to determine the end point of the brow.

Mark this point lightly with the brow pencil.

**5. Create the Tail of the Brow:**
To ensure a natural and gradual brow taper, place the straight object diagonally from the arch point to the end point.
Mark this point lightly with the brow pencil to create the tail of the brow.

**6. Double-Check Symmetry:**
Compare the markings of both brows to ensure they are symmetrical and balanced.

Adjust the markings as needed to achieve harmony between the two brows.

**7. Adjust Brow Thickness and Shape:**
Take into consideration the client's facial structure, eye shape, and personal preferences when determining the ideal brow thickness and shape.

Use the brow mapping as a guide to create a shape that complements the client's features.

**8. Finalise the Brow Design:**
Once the brow mapping is complete and both brows are symmetrical, finalise the brow design with the client's approval.

Discuss the proposed shape and make any adjustments based on the client's feedback.

**9. Hair Growth Patterns:**
Consider the client's natural hair growth patterns when creating hair strokes or shading to ensure a realistic and natural appearance.

**10. Brow Mapping Tools:**
Brow mapping tools, such as rulers with various measurements, can aid in achieving precise and balanced brow mapping.

Identifying the brow arch placement and tail position is crucial in semi-permanent brow procedures to achieve a balanced and flattering brow shape that enhances the client's facial features. Here's a step-by-step guide on how to identify the brow arch placement and tail position:

**1. Brow Starting Point:**
Begin by identifying the starting point of the brow, which is the innermost part of the brow, closest to the centre of the face.

The starting point can be determined by holding a straight object, such as a ruler or brow mapping tool, vertically along the side of the nostril and aligning it with the inner corner of the eye.

**2. Brow Arch Placement:**
To identify the brow arch placement, imagine a diagonal line from the centre of the nostril to the outer edge of the iris (the coloured part of the eye).

The highest point of the brow should align with this imaginary line, and the arch should be positioned slightly above the diagonal line.

**3. Marking the Arch Placement:**
Lightly mark the arch placement with a brow pencil or a removable marking pen to guide the semi-permanent brow procedure.

The arch point should be approximately two-thirds of the way from the starting point to the brow end point.

**4. Brow Tail Position:**
To determine the brow tail position, imagine a diagonal line from the centre of the nostril to the outer corner of the eye.

The brow tail should align with this imaginary line and extend slightly beyond it.

**5. Marking the Tail Position:**
Lightly mark the tail position with the brow pencil or marking pen, creating the endpoint of the brow.

The tail should align with the diagonal line, giving a subtle lift to the outer part of the brow.

**6. Assessing Symmetry:**
Compare the markings of both brows to ensure they are symmetrical and balanced.

Make any necessary adjustments to achieve symmetry between the two brows.

**7. Customisation for Facial Features:**
Consider the client's facial structure, eye shape, and personal preferences when determining the ideal arch and tail positions.

The brow shape should complement the client's features and create a harmonious appearance.

**8. Discuss with the Client:**
Present the proposed arch placement and tail position to the client and discuss it with them.

Take their feedback into account and make any necessary adjustments based on their preferences.

**9. Finalise the Brow Design:**
Once the arch and tail positions are agreed upon, finalise the brow design with the client's approval.

Ensure that both the client and the brow artist are satisfied with the chosen positions before proceeding with the semi-permanent brow procedure.

## Module 7: Micro blading Technique

| Semi-Permanent Brows: | Step-by-step micro blading technique, including proper pressure and hand movements. |
| --- | --- |

Micro blading is a semi-permanent brow technique that involves creating fine, hair-like strokes to mimic natural eyebrow hairs. It requires precision and attention to detail to achieve a natural and realistic appearance. Here's a step-by-step guide on the micro blading technique, including proper pressure and hand movements:

### Step 1: Preparing the Work Area:
Ensure that your work area is clean, sanitised, and well-lit.

Set up all the necessary tools and materials, including the micro blading pen, sterilised micro blades, pigments, disposable gloves, and anaesthetic cream (if used).

### Step 2: Consultation and Brow Mapping:
Begin by consulting with the client to understand their desired brow shape and preferences.

Use brow mapping techniques to measure and mark the starting point, arch, and tail position of the brows for symmetry and balance.

### Step 3: Applying Topical anaesthetic:
If the client requests it, apply a topical anaesthetic cream to the brow area to minimise discomfort during the procedure.

Allow the anaesthetic to take effect according to the manufacturer's instructions.

### Step 4: Choosing the Right Micro blade:
Select the appropriate micro blade based on the desired brow thickness and hair stroke style.

Micro blades come in various configurations, such as U-shaped, curved, or straight needles.

### Step 5: Dip and Load the Micro blade:
Dip the micro blade into the chosen pigment, ensuring that the blade's surface is evenly coated.

Wipe off any excess pigment on the edge of the pigment container.

### Step 6: Micro blading Strokes:
Hold the micro blading pen at a 45-degree angle to the skin.

Use gentle and controlled pressure to create thin, precise hair strokes that resemble natural eyebrow hairs.

Apply the strokes following the direction of hair growth, starting from the bottom of the brow and working upwards.

**Step 7: Gradual and Consistent Pressure:**
Maintain a consistent and gradual pressure as you glide the micro blade along the skin.
Avoid applying too much pressure, as it may cause the strokes to appear too thick or harsh.

**Step 8: Fill in the Brows:**
Fill in the brows by adding more hair strokes to areas where additional density is needed.

Blend the strokes seamlessly with the natural hair and existing brows, if applicable.

**Step 9: Continue the Process:**
Work your way through the entire brow, stroke by stroke, until the desired shape and fullness are achieved.

**Step 10: Check for Symmetry:**
Regularly check for symmetry between both brows, making adjustments as needed to ensure balance.

**Step 11: Aftercare and Client Instructions:**
Provide the client with aftercare instructions, including how to care for the brows during the healing process.

Schedule a follow-up appointment for a touch-up session, typically 4 to 8 weeks after the initial procedure.

Practical Skills Training Module

Semi-Permanent Brows:        Achieving fine, crisp hair strokes for natural-looking brows.

Achieving fine, crisp hair strokes is essential for creating natural-looking brows in semi-permanent brow procedures, particularly in micro blading. It requires precision, control, and attention to detail. Here are some tips to achieve fine, crisp hair strokes for natural-looking brows:

**1. Use the Right Micro blade:**
Select a micro blade with a fine needle configuration, such as a single needle or a blade with a few needles clustered together.

Finer needles allow for more precise and delicate hair strokes.

**2. Proper Blade Angle:**
Hold the micro blade at a 45-degree angle to the skin.

This angle ensures that the hair strokes are created with the right depth and mimic the natural direction of eyebrow hairs.

**3. Gentle and Controlled Pressure:**
Apply gentle and controlled pressure while making the hair strokes.

Avoid pressing too hard, as it may result in thicker and less natural-looking hair strokes.
**4. Feather-Light Strokes:**
Use feather-light strokes when creating the hair strokes.

Imagine that you are lightly grazing the surface of the skin to deposit the pigment.

**5. Follow the Direction of Hair Growth:**
Always follow the direction of natural hair growth when creating the hair strokes.

This helps the hair strokes blend seamlessly with the existing brow hairs.

**6. Vary the Length and Angle:**
To mimic the variation in natural eyebrow hairs, create hair strokes of different lengths and angles.

Avoid making the hair strokes too uniform or repetitive.

**7. Gradation of Pigment Intensity:**

Start each hair stroke with a light touch and gradually increase the pressure to achieve a gradation of pigment intensity.

This gives the hair strokes a natural-looking and dimensional appearance.

### 8. Review and Refine:
Regularly step back and review your work to ensure that the hair strokes are consistent and balanced.

Make any necessary refinements to achieve the desired result.

### 9. Work in Sections:
Divide the brow into sections and work on one section at a time.

This approach allows you to focus on creating precise and natural-looking hair strokes in each area.

### 10. Practice and Patience:
Achieving fine, crisp hair strokes takes practice and patience.

Continuously improve your micro blading technique through training and hands-on experience.

### 11. Aftercare and Touch-Up:
Provide the client with aftercare instructions to ensure proper healing of the hair strokes.

Schedule a touch-up session, typically 4 to 8 weeks after the initial procedure, to refine and enhance the hair strokes.

**Module 8: Micro shading Technique**



Micro shading, ombre, and combination techniques are popular semi-permanent brow procedures that offer different results and effects. Here's an overview of each technique:

**Micro shading:** Micro shading, also known as shading or powder brows, is a technique that involves adding soft, pixelated colour to the eyebrows. Instead of creating individual hair strokes like in micro blading, micro shading uses a stippling method to deposit pigment in a shaded or gradient effect. The result is a soft and more filled-in appearance, similar to the look achieved with brow powder or makeup. Micro shading is ideal for clients who prefer a fuller and more defined brow without the look of individual hair strokes.

**Ombre Brows:** Ombre brows, also known as gradient or powder-gradient brows, are another shading technique that creates a gradient effect from darker at the tail to lighter at the front of the brows. The technique uses a similar stippling method as micro shading but with a more pronounced gradient. The result is a soft, faded look, resembling an ombre effect. Ombre brows are suitable for clients who desire a more defined and structured brow with a seamless blend of colour.

**Combination Brows:** Combination brows, as the name suggests, combine micro blading (hair strokes) with micro shading (shading). This technique is versatile and allows brow artists to tailor the procedure to the client's preferences and facial features. The hair strokes create a natural and realistic front of the brow, while the shading adds density and definition, giving a more polished appearance. Combination brows are suitable for clients who want the best of both worlds—natural-looking hair strokes and a softly filled-in brow.

**Choosing the Right Technique:** The choice of technique depends on the client's preferences, skin type, and desired outcome. During the consultation, discuss the different options and consider factors such as the client's natural brow hair, skin condition, and daily makeup routine. Educate the client about each technique's longevity and maintenance to help them make an informed decision.

**Procedure and Aftercare:** The procedures for micro shading, ombre, and combination brows are similar in terms of consultation, brow mapping, and pigment selection. The aftercare instructions are also comparable, emphasising avoiding excessive water contact, picking at the treated area, and following the provided aftercare routine.

**Artist Expertise:** Regardless of the technique, achieving optimal results depends on the brow artist's skill, experience, and attention to detail. Continuous education and training in the latest techniques and tools are essential for delivering successful semi-permanent brow procedures.

Overall, micro shading, ombre, and combination techniques provide versatile options for clients to achieve their desired brow look, whether it's soft and natural or more defined and structured.



Micro shading is a semi-permanent brow technique that involves creating soft, pixelated shading to fill in and define the eyebrows. The shading patterns used in micro shading can vary, allowing for different effects, from soft and natural to bold and defined. Here are some shading patterns and techniques to achieve various effects in micro shading:

**1. Soft Ombre Shading:**
Soft ombre shading creates a subtle and natural gradient effect, starting with lighter shading at the front of the brows and gradually increasing in intensity towards the tails.

To achieve soft ombre shading, use a light hand pressure and a stippling motion with the micro shading tool.

Focus the shading primarily on the outer two-thirds of the brow, leaving the front (inner third) slightly lighter.

**2. Bold Ombre Shading:**
Bold ombre shading creates a more defined and structured look with a noticeable gradient effect from light to dark.

Use slightly firmer hand pressure to deposit more pigment for a bolder appearance.

The shading can extend further into the front of the brows, creating a more pronounced ombre effect.

**3. Gradient Shading:**
Gradient shading involves creating a soft and seamless transition of pigment from the top to the bottom of the brows, giving a smooth and natural appearance.

Use a combination of stippling and blending techniques to achieve the gradient effect.

The pigment density should be slightly lighter at the top of the brows and gradually increase towards the bottom.

**4. Dense and Uniform Shading:**
Dense and uniform shading creates a consistent and filled-in appearance throughout the entire brow area.

Apply firm and even pressure with the micro shading tool to deposit more pigment for a solid, non-ombre look.

**5. Hairline Blending:**

Hairline blending involves blending the micro shading at the front of the brows with individual hair strokes, creating a seamless and natural transition.

Use a fine micro blade or a single needle to create hair strokes at the front of the brows and then blend them with the shading technique.

### 6. Customising Shading Density:

Tailor the shading density based on the client's preferences and desired level of boldness.

Communicate with the client during the procedure to ensure their satisfaction with the shading intensity.

### 7. Feathering Technique:

The feathering technique involves creating delicate and soft edges around the shaded areas to enhance the natural appearance.

Use a light touch and feathering motions at the outer edges of the shading to achieve a soft and diffused look.

### 8. Gradation for Dimension:

Gradation in shading can add dimension and depth to the brows.

Gradually increase the pigment density from the front to the tail of the brows to create a 3D effect.

| Semi-Permanent Brows: | Practicing shading on artificial skin and live models. |
| --- | --- |

**Practical Skills Training Module**

**Module 9: Touch-ups and Aftercare**

Semi-Permanent Brows:    Identifying the need for touch-ups and how to perform them.

Identifying the need for touch-ups and performing them is a crucial aspect of maintaining the longevity and appearance of semi-permanent brows. Touch-ups are essential for refreshing the pigment, addressing any fading or unevenness, and ensuring that the brows continue to look their best. Here's how to identify the need for touch-ups and perform them effectively:

**1. Identifying the Need for Touch-Ups:**
Advise clients during the initial consultation that touch-ups are a standard part of the semi-permanent brow procedure.

Inform them that the initial results will soften and lighten during the healing process, and a touch-up session will be required to perfect the brows.

Suggest scheduling the touch-up session 4 to 8 weeks after the initial procedure, depending on the healing progress and the client's skin type.

**2. Assessing Pigment Retention:**
During the touch-up session, assess the client's brows to determine how much of the initial pigment has retained. Identify any areas that require additional pigment to achieve the desired colour and density.

**3. Addressing Fading and Unevenness:**
Address any areas where the pigment has faded or appears uneven.

Use the micro blading or micro shading technique to add hair strokes or shading to those areas for a seamless appearance.

**4. Customising the Brow Shape:**
Tailor the touch-up session to the client's preferences and facial features.

Make adjustments to the brow shape, if necessary, to achieve the most flattering and natural-looking result.

**5. Numbing and Preparing the Area:**
Apply a topical numbing cream to the brow area before performing the touch-up. Allow the numbing cream to take effect to minimise discomfort during the procedure.

**6. Performing the Touch-Up:**
Use the same micro blading or micro shading technique as the initial procedure to deposit pigment.

Ensure that the hand pressure and movements are consistent with the previous work for uniformity.

## 7. Gradual Layering:

Gradually layer the pigment to achieve the desired colour and intensity.

Avoid over-saturating the skin, as it may result in an unnatural appearance.

## 8. Review and Final Adjustments:

Regularly review your work during the touch-up session to ensure evenness and balance.

Make any final adjustments to achieve the best possible outcome.

## 9. Aftercare and Follow-Up:

Provide the client with aftercare instructions for the touch-up session.

Schedule a follow-up appointment to check on the healing progress and address any concerns.

## 10. Client Communication:

Communicate openly with the client throughout the touch-up session.

Address any questions or concerns they may have and ensure their satisfaction with the results.

Aftercare instructions are crucial for ensuring proper healing and colour retention after a semi-permanent brow procedure. Following these instructions helps clients achieve the best possible results and prolong the longevity of their newly enhanced brows. Here are essential aftercare instructions to provide to your clients:

**1. Keep the Area Dry:**
Avoid getting the brows wet for the first 7 to 10 days after the procedure.

Do not wash the brows directly, and try to minimise water contact during face washing or showering.

**2. Avoid Touching or Picking:**
Refrain from touching or picking at the treated area, as this can disrupt the healing process and cause pigment loss.

**3. Apply Aftercare Ointment:**
Gently apply the aftercare ointment provided by the artist to the brows as directed.

Use a clean cotton swab to apply a thin layer of the ointment 2 to 3 times a day to keep the area moisturised.

**4. Avoid Sun Exposure:**
Protect the brows from direct sunlight during the healing process.

If sun exposure is unavoidable, wear a wide-brimmed hat or use a gentle, broad-spectrum sunscreen.

**5. Avoid Excessive Sweating:**
Minimise activities that cause excessive sweating, as sweat can interfere with the pigment retention process.

Avoid intense workouts or saunas for at least 7 to 10 days after the procedure.

**6. Avoid Makeup and Skincare Products:**
Avoid applying makeup or skincare products directly to the treated area during the healing process.

Avoid using any exfoliating or peeling products near the brows.

**7. No Swimming or Soaking:**
Refrain from swimming or soaking in pools, hot tubs, or saunas during the healing period.

**8. Avoid Chemical Peels and Laser Treatments:**

Avoid chemical peels, laser treatments, and other facial treatments that may affect the brows during the healing process.

**9. Be Patient with the Healing Process:**
The colour of the brows will appear darker immediately after the procedure and will gradually soften and lighten as they heal.

Be patient and allow the brows to heal naturally.
**10. Follow-Up Appointment:**
Schedule and attend the follow-up appointment with the artist as recommended.

The touch-up session is crucial for perfecting the brows and addressing any areas that may need additional pigment.

**11. Report Any Concerns:**
If the client experiences unusual redness, swelling, itching, or signs of infection, they should contact the artist or seek medical advice promptly.

It's essential to provide clients with written aftercare instructions and verbally communicate the guidelines before they leave the appointment. Emphasise the importance of following the aftercare instructions diligently to ensure proper healing and colour retention. Clients' commitment to aftercare plays a significant role in achieving the best possible results from their semi-permanent brow procedure.

Managing common post-procedure concerns and complications is an essential aspect of providing excellent care and support to clients after a semi-permanent brow procedure. While most clients have a smooth healing process, some may experience minor issues or complications. Here's how to handle and address common concerns:

## 1. Redness and Swelling:
It is normal for the brow area to appear slightly red and swollen immediately after the procedure.

Advise clients that these symptoms should subside within a few hours to a couple of days. Applying a cold compress to the area can help reduce redness and swelling.

## 2. Itching and Dryness:
Itching and dryness may occur during the healing process.

Instruct clients to avoid scratching the area and to apply the provided aftercare ointment as directed to keep the brows moisturised.

## 3. Scabbing or Flaking:

Some clients may experience mild scabbing or flaking as the brows heal.

Remind clients not to pick or peel at the scabs, as it can affect the pigment retention and result in patchy areas.

## 4. Uneven Pigment or Fading:
Inform clients that the initial pigment may appear darker but will gradually fade and soften during the healing process.

It is common for the brows to appear slightly uneven during the initial healing phase.

Encourage clients to wait for the complete healing before evaluating the final result.

## 5. Allergic Reactions:
Although rare, some clients may experience allergic reactions to the pigment or other products used during the procedure.

If a client reports signs of an allergic reaction (severe redness, swelling, rash, or itching), instruct them to seek medical attention immediately.

## 6. Colour Dissatisfaction:
Sometimes, clients may express dissatisfaction with the colour of their brows after healing.

Remind clients that the colour will soften and become more natural as the brows heal, and it is essential to wait for the full healing before assessing the final result.

If the client is still dissatisfied after the healing process, schedule a touch-up session to make adjustments.

**7. Infection Prevention:**
Emphasise the importance of proper aftercare to prevent infection.

Instruct clients to keep the brows clean and avoid touching them with dirty hands.

**8. Follow-Up Communication:**
Stay in touch with clients after the procedure to check on their healing progress and address any concerns they may have.

Offer support and reassurance during the healing phase.

**9. Encourage Patience and Understanding:**
Managing post-procedure concerns requires patience and understanding from both the client and the artist.

Reassure clients that you are there to support them throughout the healing process.

**10. Referral to a Medical Professional:**
If any concerns or complications persist or worsen, consider referring the client to a medical professional for further evaluation and treatment.

| | |
|---|---|
| Semi-Permanent Brows: | Setting up a semi-permanent brow business, legal considerations, and insurance. |

Obtaining appropriate insurance to protect your business and clients. Here are some essential steps and considerations:

**1. Business Structure:**

Choose a suitable business structure for your semi-permanent brow business, such as a sole proprietorship, partnership, limited liability company (LLC), or corporation.

Each structure has its own legal and tax implications, so consult with a business attorney or accountant to determine the best fit for your business.

**2. Business Registration:**

Register your business with the appropriate government authorities in your country or state.

Obtain a business license or permit, if required by local regulations.

**3. Insurance:**

Obtain liability insurance for your semi-permanent brow business to protect against potential claims from clients for injuries or adverse reactions.

Consider additional coverage for property insurance, professional liability insurance, and product liability insurance.

**4. Health and Safety Regulations:**

Familiarise yourself with health and safety regulations specific to the beauty and cosmetology industry in your area.

Implement strict sanitation and Sterilisation practices to ensure a safe and hygienic environment for your clients.

**5. Compliance with Industry Standards:**

Adhere to industry standards and best practices for semi-permanent brow procedures.

Stay informed about any updates or changes in industry regulations.

**6. Licensing and Certification:**

Obtain the necessary licenses and certifications to perform semi-permanent brow procedures in your area.

Attend training programs or workshops to enhance your skills and knowledge in the field.

**7. Client Consent and Consultation:**

Develop clear and comprehensive client consent forms outlining the procedure, risks, aftercare, and possible outcomes.

Conduct thorough consultations with clients to understand their expectations and any underlying medical conditions that may affect the procedure.

### 8. Record-Keeping and Documentation:
Maintain detailed records of client information, consent forms, treatment plans, and before-and-after photos.

Keep track of all financial transactions and expenses for tax purposes.

### 9. Marketing and Advertising Compliance:
Ensure that your marketing materials and advertisements comply with truth-in-advertising regulations.

Avoid making false or misleading claims about your services.
### 10. Contracts and Policies:
Develop contracts or service agreements that outline the terms and conditions of your services, including cancellation policies and refund procedures.

### 11. Hiring and Employment Considerations:
If you plan to hire employees, familiarise yourself with employment laws and regulations in your area.

Implement fair employment practices and provide necessary training to your staff.

### 12. Continued Education and Training:
Stay up-to-date with the latest trends, techniques, and safety protocols in the semi-permanent brow industry through continued education and training.

Starting a semi-permanent brow business involves careful planning, compliance with legal requirements, and obtaining appropriate insurance coverage. Seek professional advice from business consultants, attorneys, or insurance providers to ensure that you have all the necessary legal considerations in place to run a successful and legally compliant business.

Marketing is crucial for attracting clients and building a strong clientele for your semi-permanent brow business. Here are some effective marketing strategies to help you promote your services and grow your business:

**1. Professional Branding:**
Create a professional and visually appealing brand identity, including a logo, colour scheme, and cohesive branding across all marketing materials.

Use high-quality images of your work to showcase your expertise and the results you can achieve.

**2. Social Media Presence:**
Utilise social media platforms like Instagram, Facebook, and Pinterest to showcase your before-and-after photos, client testimonials, and behind-the-scenes content.

Engage with your audience by responding to comments and direct messages promptly.

**3. Client Referral Program:**
Offer incentives to your existing clients for referring new clients to your business.

Word-of-mouth referrals can be powerful for attracting new clients.

**4. Special Offers and Promotions:**
Introduce special offers or promotions, such as discounted touch-up sessions or bundled services, to attract new clients and encourage repeat business.

**5. Collaborations and Partnerships:**
Collaborate with other beauty professionals or businesses to cross-promote each other's services.

Partner with salons, spas, or beauty events to reach a broader audience.

**6. Content Marketing:**
Create valuable and educational content related to semi-permanent brows on your website, blog, or social media.

Share tips, FAQs, and trends to position yourself as an authority in your field.

**7. Local SEO Optimisation:**
Optimise your website and online listings for local search engines to appear in relevant searches in your area.

Include keywords related to your services and location in your website content.

**8. Client Testimonials and Reviews:**
Request testimonials and reviews from satisfied clients and showcase them on your website and social media.

Positive reviews build trust and credibility with potential clients.

**9. Events and Workshops:**
Host events or workshops related to semi-permanent brows to attract potential clients and showcase your expertise.
Demonstrations and interactive sessions can create interest in your services.

**10. Networking:**
Attend beauty industry events, trade shows, and networking events to connect with potential clients and industry professionals.

Share your business cards and promotional materials at these events.

**11. Local Advertising:**
Consider advertising in local beauty or lifestyle magazines, newspapers, or online directories.

Offer special discounts or promotions for readers to encourage them to try your services.

**12. Client Loyalty Program:**
Implement a client loyalty program to reward repeat clients and encourage them to return for touch-up sessions.

Pricing, scheduling, and managing client appointments are essential aspects of running a successful semi-permanent brow business. Here's how to handle each aspect effectively:

**1. Pricing:**
Set competitive and fair pricing for your semi-permanent brow services. Consider factors such as your skill level, experience, location, and the quality of materials used.

Offer different pricing tiers based on the complexity of the procedure or the experience level of the artist.

Clearly communicate your pricing structure on your website, social media, or marketing materials.

**2. Scheduling:**
Implement an efficient scheduling system to manage client appointments. Consider using scheduling software or apps to streamline the process.

Offer various time slots to accommodate different client preferences, including evenings and weekends.

Allow sufficient time between appointments to ensure a smooth transition and provide ample time for client consultations and aftercare instructions.

**3. Booking Process:**
Offer multiple booking options, such as online booking through your website, email, or phone.

Provide clear instructions on how clients can book their appointments and any necessary pre-appointment preparations.

**4. Deposits and Cancellation Policy:**
Consider requiring a non-refundable deposit at the time of booking to secure the appointment. This helps deter last-minute cancellations or no-shows.

Implement a reasonable cancellation policy and communicate it to clients during the booking process. This policy should address any potential fees for late cancellations.

**5. Client Intake Forms:**
Have clients fill out intake forms before their appointments to gather important information, such as medical history and skin sensitivity.

These forms also help you understand the client's expectations and any specific concerns they may have.

**6. Appointment Reminders:**
Send appointment reminders to clients via email or text a day or two before their scheduled appointment.

This helps reduce no-shows and ensures that clients are prepared for their session.

**7. Efficient Consultations:**
Conduct thorough consultations with each client to understand their desired brow shape, concerns, and any specific requests.

Use this time to manage client expectations and explain the semi-permanent brow process.

**8. Organised Workspace:**
Keep your workspace clean, organised, and ready for each appointment.

Ensure that all necessary tools and materials are readily available and sanitised.

**9. Time Management:**
Allocate a specific amount of time for each appointment to maintain a consistent schedule and prevent overbooking.

Avoid rushing through appointments to ensure that each client receives the attention and care they deserve.

**10. Follow-Up and Rebooking:**
Follow up with clients after their appointments to check on their healing progress and satisfaction with the results.

Encourage clients to schedule their touch-up sessions at the appropriate time to maintain their semi-permanent brows.

## Module 11: Hands-on Practice and Assessments

Extensive hands-on practice on models under supervision.
Continuous assessments and feedback to improve skills and techniques.
Mock exams and final evaluations to test proficiency.

**Module 12: Certification and Continuing Education**
Awarding of a completion certificate to successful participants.

Encouraging ongoing education and attending advanced training courses.

Staying updated on industry trends and safety standards.

Note: The actual content and duration of the training program may vary based on the training provider and the specific techniques they teach. Always ensure that the training program is conducted by a qualified and experienced instructor to receive the best education and guidance.